The Gift Within

10 Lessons of Spiritual Awakening
and the End of Life
from a Trauma Center Chaplain

Rosemary Baron

LAYER PUBLISHING

Rosmary Baron
rosemarybaron@gmail.com

Cover Art: © Steve Sheffield, Artist, Salt Lake
Book Designer, Jim Shubin, www.bookalchemist.net

ISBN 978-1-7348251-3-8 (PaperBack)

Publisher's Cataloging-in-Publication Data

Names: Baron, Rosemary, author.
Title: The gift within : 10 lessons of spiritual awakening and the end of life from a trauma center chaplain / Rosemary Baron.
Description: Includes index. | Salt Lake City, UT: Layer Press, 2020.
Identifiers: ISBN: 978-1-7348251-3-8
Subjects: LCSH Palliative treatment—Anecdotes. | Palliative Care—Personal Narratives. | Palliative Care—Religious aspects. | Terminal care—Anecdotes. | Terminal care—Religious aspects. | Hospice care—Anecdotes. | Hospice care—Religious aspects. | Spirituality. | BISAC RELIGION / Spirituality | RELIGION / Christian Living / Death, Grief, Bereavement
Classification: LCC R726.8 .B354 2020| DDC 362.1/75—dc23

Dedicated to

Intermountain Medical Center Palliative Care Team

Dallas Aste, Operations Manager
Cory Taylor, MD
Saloni Shah, MD
Meg Randle, APRN
Melissa Wilkinson, APRN
Jeff Bowen, APRN
Treas Eddleman, LCSW
Laura Lockwood, PA-C

With love, admiration and gratitude.

Contents

Foreword

Like Rosemary Baron, I too am a chaplain. I know firsthand that ours is a much misunderstood and woefully under-valued profession in modern healthcare. Chaplains are often mistakenly thought to be well-meaning church folk whose goal is to bring patients to belief in God, sometimes on their deathbed. Chaplains are indeed people of faith. But, as Rosemary writes in her introduction, her faith functions as "integral to...my heart and desire to help patients find meaning and solace in the most difficult times of life." That desire to help people find meaning and comfort in the face of sickness and death is at the heart of healthcare chaplaincy and indeed, at the heart of the stories Rosemary so eloquently tells in this book.

The Gift Within is a treasure trove of reflections on real-life experiences Rosemary has had in her work as chaplain on a palliative care team in a large urban hospital. Palliative care is medical care offered to a patient with a life-threatening illness rather than attempting a cure. This mode of care seeks to mitigate physical pain and discomfort for the patient and to provide emotional and spiritual support to all involved in the patient's life. Palliative care is delivered by an interdisciplinary medical team of specialists working together to understand and meet the unique needs and goals of every patient. The chaplain's role is to uncover and meet people's spiritual needs, witness to the existential issues they are wrestling with, validate their doubts and fears as well as their hopes and dreams, and sometimes accompany them to the doorway of death and the threshold of life to come. This book illustrates many ways in which Rosemary has fulfilled her mission.

As the stories Rosemary recounts here illustrate, a chaplain must be vulnerable enough to be genuinely touched—even personally transformed—by the individuals under her spiritual care. Within these pages, you will join her as she wades fearlessly into the pain and suffering of the lives of people she barely knows, forging with them a bond of humanity and spirituality that never leaves her untouched. You'll be present as Rosemary witnesses healing, experiences despair, feels the pain of accompany-ing someone with a death wish, rejoices in a transformation of the spirit, discovers a soulmate, realizes she too has failed in an intimate relationship, and wonders "Why not me?" as she cares for a friend her own age who is suffering from a stroke. "We must love more and more especially those who've been damaged," this friend declares. Rosemary's life as a chaplain bears testimony to that love.

"We write to remind ourselves that we are not alone," Rosemary remembers of her writing teacher Phil Cousineau at the Connemara Writer's Retreat in Ireland. As you read the stories in *The Gift Within*, you will see that Rosemary is never alone in her work. "God is alive in my life!" she declares. Perhaps of all the gifts Rosemary has received from her work as a chaplain, this is the greatest gift of all.

—Chaplain David Pascoe

Introduction
A story without love is not worth telling.

The Gift Within: 10 Lessons of Spiritual Awakening and the End of Life from a Trauma Center Chaplain tells the stories of ten patients who have touched my chaplain heart. Everyone is the same; everyone is different. They are the same because each one experiences a life-threatening illness. They are different because each responds to their issues in relation to how they have lived their lives. From each of them I have learned: the humbling walk of their journey, their vulnerabilities, ways to address the spiritual in serious life issues, and sometimes helping them end their life's journey. Sharing the universality of the human condition in times of illness is the reason for my writing. My friend completing her degree in American Sign Language showed me the sign for soul, that spiritual force within each of us. Connecting the tips of her index finger and thumb, she gently touched her navel and slowly began a soft circular lifting motion as if a thread was extended from inside to outside. It is so with the soul of a patient. The thread of their story tells of their soul, their essence.

Preparation

When I was training to be a chaplain many years ago, each week for four quarters in Clinical Pastoral Education, I was required to write an in-depth study about a patient experience. Intense case study promoted analysis in theological, social, physical and emotional inquiry of my behavior and the behavior of patients and family members. In using that same template of writing from my chaplain formation, I found a sound expression of my work as a chaplain in exploring the profound relationship that develops with patients.

My whole life has prepared me for becoming a chaplain. My single mother stood tall in her life and expectation for each of her four children. She began every day by going to her bedroom window and thanking God for the new day and asking His blessing on her and her children. Office manager by day, sharing nightly supper together with all of us through our high school years, monitoring (and sometimes tutoring!) us in our homework, but also serving as a compassionate and active community member. Not one of us disappointed our mother, for we, too, used her as our model for excellence and service. Our sister, Barbara, is my model and our brother, Peter, is the glue that holds our family together.

My life's experience and work prepared me for daily chaplain encounters. My faith is integral to my development and life. Rooted in our home, schooled in all levels of education, lived day to day, it is that belief that keeps me centered. The commitment that my husband and I have made as we married still holds strong. Our three children have taught us the greatest lesson of life: love. As a teacher and principal, teamwork and cooperation promoted success within the classroom and school. International living, traveling, and studying enriched my life and prepared me for the cross-cultural experiences of chaplain work.

Our sister, Mary, a career high school math teacher, became a chaplain after her retirement from education. Shortly after Mary became a board-certified chaplain, she was diagnosed with stage-four ovarian cancer. That, combined with her diagnosis of Parkinson's disease twenty years before, put her chaplain work at a standstill. Her influence on me was not fully realized until after her death and my retirement from education. Our many conversations and visits in the last months of her life told me that chaplain work for her was essential even though short-lived. She discussed cases while in training. She talked about her faith and the Spirit working through her.

One example came just after her board certification. Mary was called to the maternity ward of her hospital. An unwed 16-year-old had given birth to a daughter. The grandmother of the baby wanted to have the baby adopted because of the shame it brought to the family. The young mother wanted to keep the baby but realized she could not do this by herself and needed the help of her parents. Mary was present as the chaplain: listening, reflecting, clarifying and asking if this decision could be made at another time when emotions were not so high. Both the mother and grandmother agreed to meet the following morning. Mary related that the next morning's conversation was difficult but she believed it was the work of the Spirit that became present in a decision that brought peace to the mother, grandmother and eventually the baby.

Chaplaincy

A few years passed after Mary's untimely death and I did not think of chaplaincy as a role for me. The month after my retirement, a friend asked me to come to his graduation from Clinical Pastoral Education. I sat at the graduation, listening to the experiences of the chaplains in formation and thought: *This is the work I want to do!*

I applied to the chaplain program. After soul-searching, intense self-examination, extensive reading, writing and clinical visits with patients, I completed four units of Clinical Pastoral Education. The final projects and exams complete, I became board-certified.

As chaplain on the Palliative Care team of a large urban hospital, my skills from education as well as my experiences in chaplaincy help address the needs of patients and their families. Our patients represent the community we serve. Our patients remind me of the students who attended the public schools in which I was principal. We are there to serve everyone and we use the best skills we have to do so. With a team approach, just like we used in public education, the Palliative Care team addresses the physical, social/emotional, cognitive and spiritual needs of our patients and their families. Each team member brings specific expertise. In this sacred work we are reminded that the word palliative comes from the Latin "palliare" which means "to cloak" as in the pain we relieve with each patient. Together we make each other strong to provide excellent patient care.

A dying Buddhist Vietnamese grandmother's family may have received a different dimension of care from me as I ministered to them simply because I studied in their country and was knowledgeable about their religious custom. And the grieving Hindu mother of a dying young boy from India may have gained insight from me as a result of my having experienced India in depth. Too, the family of a Muslim man who died in our hospital may have been treated more compassionately since I lived in a Muslim country. But it is not just the travel or study experiences that make the difference in chaplain work, it is my heart and desire to help patients find meaning and solace in the most difficult times of life. I know from experience of being hospitalized for two different surgeries in two different states. In one I had no chaplain visit but did receive excellent care. In the other I received daily chaplain visits and excellent care. Looking back, the hospitalization with chaplain visits gives me peace because it brought hope and belief that healing was possible.

New learning

No longer on a precise schedule as I had been in my education career, I found two areas of growth that enhanced my life and my work as a chaplain. One was art. Before retiring from education, as a middle school principal, the opportunity of learning from teachers was ever-present and inviting. While observing in classrooms, the curriculum was often engrossing. Such was the case with art. I found myself stopping in an Introduction to Art class in middle school, observing the lesson for a few minutes, being so engrossed it, and coming home at night to complete the student assignment on our kitchen table. The teacher, when I told her of my work, was so encouraging of my very elementary attempts. That study helped me to see the world in a different way. It also led to my discovery of a nationally recognized watercolorist in our community who had a place for me in her class. What joy, what an outlet, what discovery! I find that art expression helps to portray my feelings.

The second area that helped me grow is poetry. The poetry of Mary Oliver to be exact. At a conference on palliative care, I experienced the presentation by a hospice doctor who used art and poetry in describing her work with patients. So impressed with this concept, I applauded her efforts after her presentation. She said, "I have always wanted to form a group of people who would like to study poetry, particularly Mary Oliver." I said I would be interested and together we formed a group which has met monthly for the past five years. Mary Oliver tells us that we must slow down, look, listen and lose ourselves in the natural world. This new way of looking at life, at nature, at writing, has lifted me up. Part of Oliver's poem "Praying" which I use with our patients says: "Pay attention, patch a few words together...a doorway in which another voice may speak."

These areas of growth expand my spiritual life in ways I never considered because I saw the world in a different way. I had time to read, think, meditate —all of which enlarged the world for me. It is with this ongoing learning that I believe I am able to be a more effective chaplain. I have interspersed these stories with my simple art and some poetry reflections of my own. These interval art and poetry pieces help me to breathe between the heavy human stories. And they may do the same for the reader.

On first arriving as chaplain in our urban hospital, my colleague and mentor and I met with our hospital administrator. In conversation he asked how I intended to make my position known through the hospital. He suggested that writing about it for the hospital newspaper might be one way and hoped we would visit the editor of the newspaper as we left his office. The editor invited me to write about chaplain work and other stories with a universal appeal for a monthly contribution to the paper. With his continued encouragement and flawless editing, I have been able to make that contribution to our hospital.

Phil Cousineau, internationally recognized writer, teacher and facilitator of Connemara Writer's Workshop, Renvyle House, Galway, Ireland, helped me to begin to think like a writer and realize that what I

had to say was important. Notes from his insightful
teaching include:

- We write to remind ourselves that we are not
  alone.
- The soul lies naked in the details.
- How can I help make this sacred?
- What would you write if you weren't afraid?
- We secretly long to read about the inner struggle
  of others.
- Simplicity is the ultimate sophistication.
- Don't ask too many questions; just listen.
- If you don't love it, it won't work.

These notes and many others from this workshop
have guided me in this writing. Our hospital writer
and editor, Rich Nash, continuously encouraged me
and edited this work. With my simple art and poetic
reflections of my own, the patient stories settle.

Becoming

Many people, when hearing of my work with the
sick and dying, respond with, "Oh, I could never do
that. It is too hard, too sad, too difficult." They are
right. This work can be hard, sad, difficult. But the
gifts I receive in return are always worth it.

The first role of the chaplain is to be present.
That often includes listening, reflecting, being silent,
being with someone. Really, isn't that what we all

want from anyone who comes into our lives? In our hurried world the simplest but most profound interactions are often overlooked. Yet those actions are the essence of who we are as humans: being there for one another. Meister Eckhart expresses it like this:

> You will know
> when God has taken up residence in your heart.
> How?
> Your spirit will move with swiftness and
>   striving;
> you won't be caught just thinking about things.
> For this God of ours is not a God of thoughts
> so much as a God alive.

So it is with me. God is alive in my life! And in the stories of the patients in the pages that follow, God is alive in the lives of each of these people.

I wrote this book to tell of the lessons I learned from ten patients. These are the real lessons of life, the lessons that give us vision, strength, affirmation of our very existence. I wrote this book because these lessons are often left untold, hidden. They are often regarded as too difficult, too unsavory to talk about. Yes, they are difficult. But they are the sacred times of people's lives and we long for these lessons to be told. They are lessons of the heart. Not one of us will be untouched by the illness or end of life of someone we love and care for. These real stories provide profound insight, opened my heart, lifted me up and encouraged me to share them. I hope they will open your heart, lift your spirit and share your responses with others.

       —Rosemary Baron
        Salt Lake City, Utah
        Autumn 2020

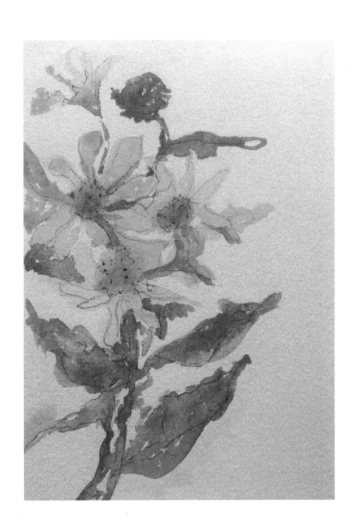

Whose Flowers Are These?

Whose flowers are these?
    prickly circled centers
    translucent yellow slivers
    sappy knotted buds
    furry pointed leaves
        The earth's?
        The sun's?
        Mine in a crystal vase?
Whose are they?
The gift of the Giver.

Tim
"My mother sent you to me."

"You don't know me. I'm a chaplain from Montana. My name is Susan. I'm the aunt of a patient in your hospital named Tim. He tried to kill himself. He's my nephew and I'm calling to ask you to pray with him."

The chaplain on the other end of the phone line continued. The mother of her nephew — her sister — had died eight months ago. Susan said her death was more difficult for Tim than for anyone else in the family. The mother was Catholic but Susan wasn't sure if Tim was practicing any faith. Susan said she'd like to hear how Tim was doing, and if I visited him, would I ask his permission to call and tell her about our visit?

I agreed to visit Tim.

Immediately I noticed how handsome he was —tawny skin, black hair, slight build, the right side of his face angular. His left eye was swollen closed, his chin was lifted up in stitches, his mouth wired shut to support the jaw. A tracheostomy tube, feeding tube, and IVs helped paint the severity of his medical condition with his attempt to take his own life. In bed, Tim was shirtless, the head of the bed raised slightly.

I introduced myself and told Tim how I came to see him.

He nodded his understanding when I told him about his aunt's call and said that I, too, was a chaplain. I told him I knew about his attempt to take his life and about his mother's death just months before.

He nodded again.

I asked him about his work. He looked to his aide who was on the periphery of the room and the aide gave Tim a clipboard and pencil. As he leaned forward I noticed angel wings lightly tattooed on his back. On the clipboard he wrote, "Construction. Fired." I asked how he made a living and he wrote, "Sell drugs."

"Involved with the law?" I continued.

"Yes. Jail." Tears began to flow. Then he wrote, "My mother sent you to me."

"Your mother?"

He wrote, "Yes — she is like you."

I asked what his mother would want for him and he wrote, "Get a job and take care of myself."

The continued verbal and written exchange made clear that Tim could stay with his sister if he was clean and had a job. I asked about his faith. "Catholic," he wrote. "No church." I explained we had a priest who visited Catholic patients in our hospital and asked if he'd like a visit. He nodded and I stepped outside to make the call then confirmed with Tim that the priest would visit in an hour. I told Tim I'd visit him again.

I felt breathless after that first visit, surprised that he communicated so openly with me on his clipboard. I was glad he'd agreed to see a priest although he was not active in his religion. I wondered if the angel wings tattooed on his back perhaps reflected a belief that angels were watching over him. I remember taking several deep breaths after I left Tim's room, the energy sucked from me. I needed to reenergize, regain balance — so great was the sadness of this young man, and his sadness made me sad.

I called Susan, told her of my conversation with Tim and the priest who would visit him that day. Susan thanked me and said she hoped I could visit Tim again. She said it was significant to think that he said his mother sent me to him. Susan told me Tim had a very supportive father, two sisters, and a brother — all of whom wanted to help him.

The link from chaplain to chaplain affirmed the trust that's often present in spiritual work. It seemed to validate my work with Tim. Though I don't know exactly how divine intervention works, the very fact that Tim thought his mother sent me to him through his aunt speaks to the spiritual energy that is alive between beings.

Tim stayed in my mind that evening. I prayed for him and tried to connect in my mind with his mother; I told her about my visit with Tim and how he'd connected her to me. I trusted God my communication to her would be made.

The next day I saw that Tim's trach was removed. He tried to speak but his jaw was still wired shut. He wrote on the clipboard that the priest's visit was good and he received the Blessing of the Sick sacrament. Tim said the priest told him that though he was very sick, healing was possible but he had a lot of work to do.

Tim was anxious and wanted to leave the hospital. I shared my understanding that he wasn't able to leave; he needed additional help. He waved me off. I said nothing for a long time and Tim looked away. Eventually I asked if I could pray with him and he nodded. I asked if I could hold his hands and he nodded again. I prayed for the healing presence of God to be with him in mind, body, and spirit. I united us to his mother in heaven; I asked for her to pray for Tim.

As I prayed, I noticed that Tim became less tense, teared up, and put his head down lower than at the beginning of prayer. At the end of my prayer, I said two Catholic prayers. When I finished, Tim gasped through his wired jaw said, "Thank you." He stood up. I stood up. He was crying and hugged me and I hugged him.

The next day I received a message from Tim's aide asking if I could drop by to meet Tim's father. Tim, still connected to IVs, sat next to me on a couch near the large window in his room. His father, Sam, sat across from us. Sam said Tim wanted him to meet me because he thought his wife had somehow inspired me to visit Tim.

Sam told me the story of his wife and Tim's mother — the significant woman in both of their lives. She was bigger than life, he said, and loved her children, especially Tim, and was totally involved in their lives. She had been a five-year survivor of ovarian cancer and was declared cancer-free and everyone rejoiced. Then, a year ago, the cancer returned with a vengeance. She did everything to fight the rage inside her. She was in constant pain. She took pain meds. Sam said some think she intentionally took an overdose to end the pain. He couldn't accept that explanation in his own mind. But the fact was, she was dead and pain meds were the reason.

"Tim," Sam said, "is diagnosed as bipolar. He takes medication sporadically. He's depressed, cannot focus, and is disconnected from life." Tim didn't respond but looked out the window as his dad described him.

Sam continued. Tim, who was living with his father, left home in a rage the night he attempted to take his life. Sam wasn't aware until the following morning that his handgun was gone. He immediately contacted the police to alert them of the possibility of Tim doing harm to himself. Almost immediately Sam knew Tim was in the hospital. Coincidentally, Tim was in the exact ICU room where his mother had been. Though she didn't die in the room, the same placement of mother and son spooked his daughters, Sam said.

The most important thing now, according to this father, was to support Tim in getting better. Though not sure of the route, he knew Tim needed a lot of help — physically, mentally, spiritually.

Sam said Tim told him I'd prayed with him and asked me to pray with both of them. I asked what their intention for prayer would be and Sam said, "Make Tim whole again." We joined hands, heads bowed in prayer and tears flowing. In this visit, even though Tim was physically with us, he appeared distant and detached. He stared off into space and looked downcast.

The next days brought physical improvement to Tim. But he was anxious; he was upset he couldn't talk and continued to slur his words through his wired jaw. He moved like a caged animal in the room. The hospital required that he have an assistant with him 24/7 and Tim resisted his sitter. Before he had welcomed my visit, but now he was edgy. I was brief and with his permission, prayed briefly.

The following day I visited Tim and found him wrapped in a heavy blanket, lying on the couch facing the window. I quietly greeted him. He didn't look at me, said nothing, then waved me away. I told him I'd hold him in my best thoughts and prayers that day and left his room.

Two days later, Tim's nurse told me he'd be moved that afternoon to another hospital for a psychiatric evaluation. She advised me to go see him because his sisters were with him.

When I visited, Tim's two beautiful sisters told me how much they loved him and wanted him to get better. Tim sat on the couch by the window, dis-engaged in the conversation. Tim's sisters asked me to pray for him before he left. I asked Tim if I could pray and he patted the seat on the couch next to him. I sat next to him and the girls sat across from us. We held hands in a circle and prayed for Tim in this new facility, for his mother to be with him in his journey, and for his good response to his new treatment. When we finished, we all stood, crying, and we hugged each other.

I don't know what happened to Tim since then. I don't know how he's doing. But as a chaplain, as a human being, Tim stayed with me in my mind and in my heart.

I believe we are where we are meant to be. I was meant to be with Tim. In the spiritual realm I believe there are no coincidences.

The call to me from Tim's aunt was not a coincidence.

Tim's belief that his mother sent me to him was not a coincidence.

The visit from our hospital priest was not a coincidence.

Meeting Tim's family and praying together was not a coincidence.

Tim's mother dying of ovarian cancer — which is the same disease that claimed the life of my sister — was not a coincidence.

The providence of God, I believe, was at work in Tim's life.

Tim trusted me and accepted me even though he was affected by his mental illness and drug addiction. There was a spiritual dimension of Tim that was ever-present and alive in him. It may have been buried when he attempted to take his own life, but it was alive in the encounters between us. Even when he waved me off, dismissing me, I sensed his spiritual dimension in his unrest.

I did what hospital chaplains do. I was present. I prayed with and for Tim. I listened, reflected, clarified. Sometimes I offer to remember patients in continued prayer after they leave my hospital, and Tim was one of those patients. I keep a list of many patients and sometimes refer to it before I pray. Tim often comes to my mind. I commend him to his mother and my sister and request their prayers for him. I remember his family and pray for their continued support.

Tim will always be in my heart and in my prayers. Though I may never see him again, I trust that our continued spiritual connection will help him. I continue to hope the angel wings tattooed on his back are a symbol of real angels who are protecting him in his journey.

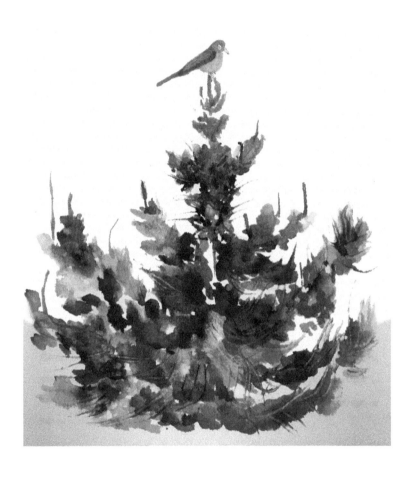

Soft Dawn Light

through open bedroom window

    five chirps
    five chirps
    five chirps
    six chirps

robin chirps me back to sleep

Donald
"I don't talk to God, but I swear at him once in a while."

*I*n a darkened unlit hospital room, gray from the rainy day, Donald sat in his bed, hunched over in a gray heap, dozing. He woke when I said his name. I sat on a stool next to his bed. He spoke softly.

His story was singular. He lived alone, worked alone as an accountant, had no friends. His brother brought Donald from California to Utah for medical care and to live permanently near the only family he had. Lung and breathing issues brought him to our hospital. He would move that afternoon to a senior care facility.

I told Donald I was a chaplain. I asked what priorities were most important to him. He said being close to his brother. When I asked if he'd like me to pray with him, he said, "I guess you could." Though he has no religion, he said he believed in God. I asked if he talked to God and he replied, "No, but I swear at him once in a while."

I asked if I could hold his hands while we prayed and he extended his hands towards me. He said, "The last time I remember praying was in a Catholic ceremony in Vietnam." Tears flowed; he sobbed. I was silent, then questioned, "Vietnam?"

His story unfolded.

"Yes. A long time ago. 1966."

"What was it you did?"

"Drove a big Caterpillar and bulldozer, making inroads in the jungle. Slept in ditches for the whole year. When we needed parts I became good at 'acquisitions.'" He paused and smiled to himself. "You did what you had to do to keep those machines going. I came home alive."

"And why the tears?" I asked.

"Because of the hatred."

"Hatred?"

"For the American soldier. We were hated when we came home. We were told not to wear our uniforms or we'd be scorned and ridiculed."

"That's what you were told?"

"Yes, that's the way it was."

We talked briefly about his experience, his feelings of isolation and lack of gratitude for his service. Finally, almost dismissively, he said, "It was a long time ago."

I asked if he had intentions to pray. He said, "No, you know how to do this."

Continuing to hold his hands, I prayed in thanks for Donald and 'lifted him up" to God asking for His blessing on Donald's life. I thanked God for Donald's service and for the thousands of service men and women who protect our nation. I asked God to keep Donald close to Him. I prayed for his protection and good response to medical treatment. I prayed for his peace.

Donald continued to cry during prayer. When I finished, he said, "Thank you. That was a long time ago. Thank you for your visit. It was just what I needed."

In debriefing about this visit, our palliative care social worker suggested my being Donald's age and a woman may have held special meaning for him and spurred his tears and emotions of lost relationships in his life. Our social worker also told me how much Donald's brother emphasized in their phone call about how alone Donald had been all of his adult life. I thought of Mother Teresa's statement about loneliness being the greatest disease in our world.

Though I may never see Donald again, his story stuck with me and jolted me into my memories of Vietnam in the late 60s and my trip there 40 years later.

In the 70s my husband and I lived on Guam, which was home to Air Force and Navy bases. The constant drone of B52 bombers landing after dropping bombs on Vietnam was ever present. Constant talk and disagreement about American involvement in the war became a daily conversation among our island friends and co-workers. We had very limited access to TV, so we didn't have any information about on-the-ground war activity like stateside Americans had. The Vietnam War was always present — but distant from us.

Years later, I received a Fulbright Award from the U.S. Department of State to study in Vietnam, and I traveled there with a dozen American educators in 2004. We experienced this beautiful S-shaped country from north to south in an effort to understand its history, culture, and traditions so we could share our new learning when we returned to our own educational settings. Our hosts put their best foot forward and ensured we experienced the finest.

One day as we toured Danang, we were warned not to step off the path, since there were still mines that hadn't been deactivated. Later we learned of the Chu Chi Tunnels, a sophisticated labyrinth of underground tunnels designed by the Viet Cong to snare US soldiers. The stories about torture of our men were horrific.

At one point a tunnel was expanded to fit American bodies, which were much larger than the Vietnamese. Those in our group who wanted to experience the descent and elbow-crawl through the pitch-dark tunnel for 1,500 feet were invited to do so. In some small way this helped me to understand how our soldiers began in a tunnel that would fit their body only to come to a point where they were trapped and killed by the Viet Cong. As I elbowed my way along this tunnel, with its sides so close overhead and around my body, the dirt embedded in my skin and clothes. When I reached the end of the tunnel, I had a hotel with a hot bath to welcome me at the end of the day. Our soldiers had death.

I thought of Danang and Chu Chi in relation to Donald and how he must have suffered as he served our nation and worked to bring the hope of peace to Vietnam. I saw the vast disparities as he slept in ditches for a year and I in comfortable beds on a first-class learning trip. The disparages of life — his single and alone, mine full of human engagement and experience. His return to the states was hidden; mine was hailed. I mentioned none of my experience in Vietnam to Donald. It seemed irrelevant in comparison to his service to our country.

As I thought about my visit with Donald, I appreciated our interaction and hoped my ministrations were appropriate. But he didn't leave my thoughts. I thought about how alone, disconnected, and unappreciated he must have felt all these years. Having his brother reach out to him and invite him to be close made an important difference in Donald's life. Holding his hands, seeing his tears, his sincerity — those human connections were unforgettable in my brief encounter with Donald. He was human enough to share his vulnerability with one he never met and would not see again. My life was transformed by this interaction. I continue to pray for Donald, to "lift him up to God" in thanksgiving for his gift to our country and to me.

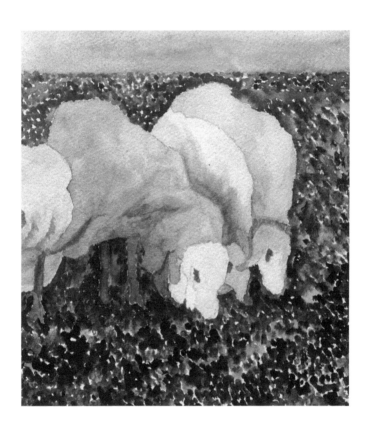

Sheep

Sheep do what sheep do.
    Eat grass, eat grass.
    Make wool, make meat.
    Stay calm.
    Keep each other company at night
    on the Connemara coast
    they call home,
        listening to the steady
        swooshing in
        sliding out
        of waves
    the eternal song of nature
    on the rocks,
  on the stones
that formed us.

Pollo
"Anytime God wants to take me, I'm ready."

Pollo, who'd been brought to the ED by his adult children, was diagnosed with kidney failure. He was our patient for the next six weeks as he received dialysis to keep him alive. He'd been blinded a few years before with complications from diabetes, but that didn't affect his disposition. He was mild-mannered, receptive to treatment, and kind to every person who entered his room.

He'd crossed the border from Mexico into the U.S. at age 13 and became and remained an undocumented worker, gainfully employed all of his adult life until the previous few months before his hospital admission. He wasn't entitled to US government assistance because he was undocumented. His children hoped to be able to buy insurance coverage during open enrollment, but ultimately this wasn't within their financial reach. Kidney transplant wasn't an option as Pollo had no insurance. Continued dialysis was financially prohibitive.

Pollo's case was brought to my hospital's Bio-ethics Committee with the plea that he continue on dialysis at no charge. But based on precedents set at the national level, his dialysis couldn't be continued without payment because of his undoc-umented status. Returning to his home village in Mexico would be foreign to him since he hadn't been there for 50 years. The village was far from medical help and transportation was non-existent.

I visited Pollo numerous times in six weeks, and two of our visits tell the story of who he really is. The first is about a walk. One day I asked Pollo if there was anything I could do to help him. He said, "You mentioned it is a beautiful day. Could you go for a walk with me?" I checked with his nurse, who said a walk would probably help him more than anything, then asked a colleague to join me.

We helped Pollo put on his shoes, and we left his room with him in in his blue hospital gown and pants. I asked him to take our arms so he'd be safe. As soon as he took my arm, he said, "Now I know how tall you are." We laughed because I was easily six inches taller than he.

As soon as we stepped outside, Pollo lifted his face to the sun and said how warm, enveloping, and alive it made him feel. We stopped in silence to listen to the fountains and waterfalls in our campus's healing gardens. A mild breeze brought a fresh new life to our adventure. With sure steps, we continued walking, mostly in easy silence. In forty-five minutes, we walked the perimeter of our large hospital campus.

On reentering the hospital, Pollo thanked us and said, "This is the best day of my whole hospital stay. I feel so alive, like there is nothing wrong with me." At that moment, there was nothing wrong with Pollo. He seemed near perfect in his contentment.

Nature was alive and well during our walk. The warmth of the sun reminded me of Antonio Machado's poem, "Last Night As I Was Sleeping," which says in part: "The fiery sun was burning inside my heart; it gave light and brought tears to my eyes." The water we'd seen brought an image from the same poem — "A spring is breaking out inside my heart...water of a new life that I have never drunk." The soft wind was like the spirit moving inside each of us as we breathed fresh air and enjoyed nature.

My second especially memorable visit with Pollo came in response to a request from a local TV station that wanted to report on the work of the hospital chaplain. They said the piece would be more real if it included a patient's perspective. I asked Pollo if he'd be interested in telling his story. He readily agreed, saying, "If I can help someone understand, then I am ready."

The coverage told how Pollo had come to the hospital and reported that he'd die in about ten days if he discontinued dialysis. "Right here in the hospital they found that my kidneys failed," said Pollo on film. "Rosemary helped me to talk about this. She listened and then repeated what I said." He continued, "She prayed with me in every visit and that really helped me."

Then Pollo clearly said, "If you are ready to go, you are ready to go. Anytime God wants to take me, I'm ready."

Watching the news story was eye-opening to his family. Never had he been so clear in sharing his expectations. His family had resisted the idea that Pollo should stop dialysis. But there was no financial way they or Pollo could maintain his treatment. The TV piece helped him convey his decision and his family honored his choice. A few days later Pollo went to live in his daughter's home on hospice care. Nine days later his daughter called me to say Pollo had died peacefully.

Pollo profoundly affected me as a chaplain. In prayer we talked not only to God, but to each other. We spoke from our hearts. Sometimes Pollo would ask if he could pray in Spanish, his first language. I welcomed it and learned from him, not because I understood every word, but because I understood his message through his sacred tone.

Our friendship left me with existential questions: Why him and not me? Why do I have the financial means he doesn't have? Why is my health so perfect and his is not? Why did God desire that we two meet? But the things that made us different made no sense when I considered Pollo's gift of himself in mind, body, and spirit to me and to his family. He simply was Pollo. He knew he would die. He accepted it.

Dialysis means cleansing the body and achieving balance. As I look at our friendship, perhaps his dialysis was a metaphor for my own cleansing and balance. I became a better chaplain because the divine light that flowed into Pollo flowed into me. I continue to carry it with me.

I considered Pollo anam cara — a soul friend — as John O'Donohue describes in his book of the same name. "Anam cara brings integration and healing...it gradually refines your sensibility and transforms your way of being in the world. It is a sacred experience," says O'Donohue.

The gift Pollo gave to his family was communion with God. "When He is ready, I am ready."

His peaceful acceptance of his death was so different from the choices of some patients who insist that everything be done with artificial trappings to keep them alive. Pollo's seamless passing was a gift of peace and love for his children, and it showed how the gift of the Spirit was alive in his life.

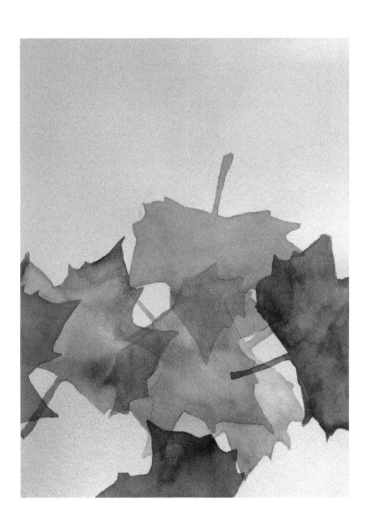

Maple Leaf

Soft deep snow
fallen in the night
      called my husband.

      Clad in snow-shoveling clothes
      he ventured out.

Moments later
      he appeared inside
      the back door
      calling my name.

"Look what I found on the doorstep
away from the snow.
I knew you'd love it."

His heavy gloved hand
presented
a perfect
deep gold-colored
maple leaf.

For one usually so sober,
      his joy at presenting it to me –
      like a precious gift
      because it was –
      left me awestruck
      with love.

An Immigrant Woman
"My husband is dying and I never loved him enough..."

The cardiologist called me. "I need your help. Not with a patient, but the wife of a patient." The story unfolded. They were immigrants who'd worked hard to pay for excellent educations for their three children. The husband suffered a massive stroke and wouldn't live.

I entered the patient's room to see the wife thrown over the chest of her husband. Her short, stout figure showed a disheveled dress and sweater, her short, white-streaked auburn hair matted to her head. Her sobbing and crying took my breath away; her anguish and sadness were intense. The unresponsive husband, his face misshapened by an intubation tube, heaved his chest with medically induced forced air.

I went to the wife and gently placed my hands on the back of her shoulders and remained silent. After a time she turned and threw herself at me. I hugged her, cried with her; we were two women sharing the universal sorrow of loss. Her emotional body heat from crying, her warm dampness, became mine in our embrace. We stayed like that for a time, then her crying slowed and her gasping lessened. Finally with one big inhale, she moved away from me, looked at me, and began to breathe normally as if in acceptance. Slowly she released her clinging and we sat in chairs close to her husband's bedside.

"I never loved him enough," she said. " Now he is gone from me." Emotionally wrenched, this woman wove the story of their lives and their immigration to the U.S. Though they worked as professionals in their Eastern European country, their professional credentials weren't accepted in this country. Each of them worked three jobs to provide for their children's educational and professional success. The children did succeed; they became doctors of different specialties. "But what did this matter?" she asked. "My husband is dying and I never loved him enough. We were always too busy. Now it's too late."

Suddenly she asked, "Are you Orthodox?"

"No."

"Believe in God?"

"Yes."

"Pray?"

"For what should we pray?"

"That my husband knows I love him, that he is at peace with God."

Holding hands, we prayed, her intensity signaled by her wet hands and wet eyes.

Then I said to her, "As long as your husband is breathing, he will hear you."

She looked at me in disbelief, but went to her husband's bed, leaned closely to his ear, and spoke softly to him. I didn't hear what she said. I didn't need to. She spoke with her heart.

That afternoon the three children gathered with their mother as their husband and father was disconnected from life support and died. After a long, deep breath, the wife seemingly acknowledged the end of her shared life with her husband and the beginning of her life without him.

This brief encounter with this woman, who I will never see again, has had a profound effect on me.

On a human level, I shared the wife's sadness. I, too, have never loved my husband enough. I, too, was flushed with emotion, warmed by this close physical and spiritual encounter. My tears were not only for this wife and her loss, but for my loss of a more meaningful relationship with my husband.

Our extreme political and social differences separate my husband and me. My psychological, intellectual, and emotional needs are often met outside of our marriage. I daily turn to God to ask for the grace to show me the way. In our faith tradition there is little choice but to remain in our marriage. In my husband's black-and-white world and my gray world, we have worked to find a balance, a way of living peaceful lives, a way of holding our differences at bay. I recognize there will never be communion between us in many perceptions and thoughts. I accept what is. But it does not mean I am unhappy. But really, what is happiness? Perhaps it is in recognizing and maintaining the commitment we made at our wedding.

I haven't told my husband I love him when he washes the floor, does my laundry, does the dishes, empties the trash, or carries my luggage. I am good at complaining that he doesn't "get" the message of a movie, won't read a book I love, or spaces out at conversations that have a liberal intellectual bent. He often asks me to look at the numbers of the daily stock reports and my eyes glaze over. His love of gardening and skill at growing the vegetables we eat is admirable, but it's not my love as it is his. But I love the vegetables he tends and harvests.

My husband and I appreciate our differences, our connections with people and continents, the sacredness of our union, and our recognition that there is more than one answer, that we are human. We find differences in our lives, accept some and argue over others, but when we merge together on the big issues of life then we are one. In understanding that, it is enough to realize that I love him.

Day to day there is balance. Yes! I will tell him that. We balance each other. I love him enough to appreciate that. That is my lesson from the immigrant woman!

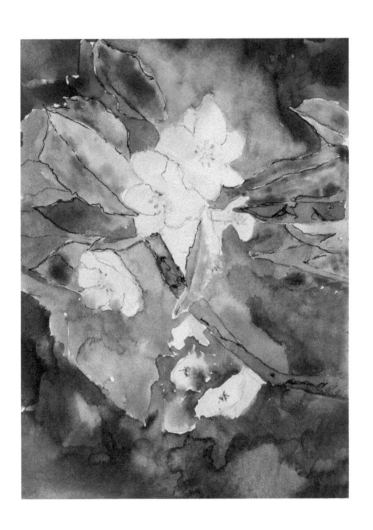

Mary's Tree

Mary's tree.
A mere sapling when first discovered.
The place my husband and I stopped on our nightly walks.
> Walks to shake out our sadness.
> Walks to talk it out.
> Walks to process life.

My sister Mary, diagnosed with ovarian cancer,
> intensified by 20 years of Parkinson's Disease

Too young for a killer combination.

The perfect person—
> selfless
> giving
> exemplary
> wife
> mother
> sister
> teacher
> community member
> chaplain.

We joined in her life—a life lived fully to the end.
We joined her in death, sending her to God.

Mary's tree—
> our stopping place
> a place of holiness
> a place of nature
> a place to find God
> a place of prayer
> a place of remembering.

Michael

"I wonder what happens between life and death?"

*I*f there was ever a patient who loved Jesus, it was Michael. Long before his car accident, he composed music and lyrics and published them on You Tube. A stanza of one song tells of his belief:

> You are greatest when I am weakest.
> You are strongest when I'm small.
> And if I lived my life without You,
> I would have no life at all.
> I would have no life at all.

For the last five months of his life, Michael was in and out of our hospital. I was his chaplain. A car accident five years before pushed the engine of his car onto Michael's lap. He was left a paraplegic with extensive upper torso damage. For these years he received medical treatment in hospitals and care centers but there would be no return to health or to home. His deterioration included an inability to stand or walk, extensive bed sores, respiratory failure, and general failure to thrive. Michael was "trached," which meant he couldn't talk without holding the stopper over the tracheostomy tube implanted in his throat. Most often, he wrote on a clipboard. Sometimes he mouthed words. He was our hospital patient when he was referred for palliative care. Despite his physical limitations, his handsome face and wide smile were engaging.

A complex man, Michael asked existential questions, expressed himself artistically, acknowledged his emotions and vulnerabilities, welcomed prayer, and reached out to people who could, in his words, "lift him up."

When I initially met Michael, he told me about himself and said he wrote music. When I told him I'd Google him, he wrote the names of one of his songs and the performing group. With his permission, I prayed for him and asked that he'd have God's healing presence in mind, body and spirit.

The following day I showed Michael what I'd found about his musical group and his website on my phone. He laughed. His lyrics said:

> Your face
> Your presence
> You are all I seek.

My Heart
Without you.
You are all I seek.

It's clear
No fear now.
You listen when I pray.

It's clear.
I see now.
The part you play.

With you,
No fear now.
You listen when I pray.

"Any formal music training?" I asked.

"No." He pointed to his head and heart.

I said, "It came from within — this acknowl-edgement of God and how you see Him?"

He nodded his head "Yes." And then he began to tear up.

"Why the tears?" I asked.

He gave no response.

I waited a long time, then I asked him what I could do for him.

He wrote, "Please call my pastor and ask him to visit." He wrote the name of the pastor and the name of the church he attended. I prayed with Michael and he thanked me.

The following day he said that even though he believes in God and talks to Him, he is so sad within himself. I acknowledged his sadness. His life was ending with an abrupt turn of events over which he had no control except how he chooses to respond. He was waiting for death when he should be at the apex of his life. He reflected on these thoughts for a long, silent time. He asked me to pray that he wouldn't be so sad.

A few days later Michael was so happy to tell me his pastor had visited him. Michael scribbled notes that said his pastor didn't know the severity of his condition and was surprised by how much he'd deteriorated since their previous visit some time ago. His pastor promised to visit frequently, which made Michael very happy.

In the next weeks Michael moved from the hospital to a care center, then back to the hospital. His reflections were profound. One day he wrote, "My life is ending. I am coming to terms with it." Then he asked, "I wonder what happens between life and death. Do you know?"

I told him I didn't entirely know, but for those who believe in the promise of eternal life, our hope is that we'll enter heaven as promised. I told him of a poem that talks about finding God in many places, even at the end of life. It is Antonio Machado's "Last Night as I Was Sleeping..." I asked if he'd like to hear it and he did. The final line says, "And listen at the shores of the great silence."

I asked Michael what the "great silence" meant to him and he said, "Death and what comes after." He was silent, pensive. I asked, "Is that enough reflection for one day?" He smiled. I prayed with Michael that he'd know more about the "shores of the great silence." Then he asked me to call a Christian Life Center he had attended. There was man there he'd like to see.

At my next visit, Michael was re-situated in a chair. Though it was a difficult process to lift him on a pulley, the staff had moved him in an attempt to make him more comfortable. "A change of scene," he mouthed. When the staff left, Michael mouthed, "I am so sad....I am going to die. The doctor told me a few weeks to a month." I asked what he thought about that news. He pointed upward with his hands. Then he wrote, "It's in God's hands."

I told him he was right. I asked what he really wanted at this time and he said, "Peace." Then he looked at the ceiling, extended his hands and mouthed, "And for His will."

Michael cried. In silence I held his hand for a long time. I thought of Psalm 139 and softly said a few lines, "Lord, You search me and You know me, You know when I sit and when I stand, You understand my thoughts from afar." Michael and I continued to hold hands until he was peaceful. He opened his eyes and thanked me.

Then he mouthed, "I talk to my parents. I ask for help. I think they hear me." Knowing that his parents had died when they were fairly young, I asked how he felt in these talks. He mouthed, "Good. They know me." Then he showed me his clipboard writing:

> To surrender to God and to let go. I feel the effects of being sick but also alive and the two don't ever meet. I have to accept the inevitable fact that God has not done this to me but allowed it to be this way. He will bring me home to Him. I struggle with the outright dying. Maybe antibiotics can give me a little more time. I want that. Given that, the rest depends on God. He alone knows the hour of my death. What a GIFT! God is gracious on every end, faithful at every point. Whom shall I fear?

The profound message of his writing affirmed to me again the depth of Michael's belief in God. I told him he was the one who'd voiced our shared prayer that day. He smiled and cried as I praised his writing.

—⚬⚬— —⚬⚬— —⚬⚬— —⚬⚬—

In my next visit, Michael was again in a chair with his legs extended. He was writing furiously and held it up for me to see. The top of the page said, "Last Will and Testament." He pointed to a few of the names and mouthed descriptions of them. He was unsure of what to include in this will, and I suggested we Google a format on his iPad. He did and found samples that would guide him. I suggested that his social worker could coordinate his work as they talked with Michael's cousin, who held his medical power of attorney. He said he had a life insurance policy that would be enough to enhance the lives of his brother, niece, and nephew. He liked being able to share.

I knew Michael was being moved to a care center and I wouldn't see him on a continuing basis. I told him I'd be away for a few weeks but promised I'd pray for him every day. He mouthed, "I will miss you." I prayed with him. He cried and mouthed, "You are my friend." And I told him he would always be my friend. He asked me to visit him in his care center when I returned and I told him I would.

Twenty days later I visited Michael. As he looked at me from his bed, he smiled and then began to cry.

I held his hands and hugged him and said, "I really missed you." He, too, said the same. Then he mouthed, "Where have you been?" I told him I was in the Holy Land. He immediately mouthed, "Tell me about Jerusalem."

I told him about the Eternal City, the variety of powerful forces there, including the three religions that consider it holy — Judaism, Christianity, and Islam, each with their own beliefs and points of view, all living in relative harmony. I told Michael that in every church I entered, I prayed for him and often lit a candle, which is customary when praying for special intentions. I gave him an olive wood palm cross from the Holy Land. He held it to his heart and began to cry. He mouthed, "I like how it feels."

The next weeks Michael came back to the hospital again. Doctors told him he was on comfort care and hospital visits wouldn't help his condition. Finally, Michael was moved to a care center. In our visit, he showed me the lyrics of a song he was writing:

> The only road to Jesus,
> The only way He sees us,
> Is alone.
> And He will never leave us,
> And He will never fail us,
> The only road to Jesus
> Is alone.

I asked him what he was thinking about and he said, "To surrender to God and let go."

—ⱳ— —ⱳ— —ⱳ— —ⱳ—

One day soon after, Michael was drawing with colored pencils. He had drawn flowers and told me, "For you." I thanked him. Then he showed me another drawing of a man — himself — above a cross, which was surrounded by several broken hearts in a pile. The figure, he explained, was throwing his broken heart to the cross in order to be made whole. Then he showed me a full-page reflection on dying and asking God and Jesus to forgive him for anything he had done in his life that would keep him from God. I read it silently, then quietly reflected on it with Michael. He smiled as if saying I understood his intention. I prayed with Michael, and voiced his reflection of his broken heart and his need to be healed.

In my next visit, I asked Michael what we should pray for and he whispered, "Faith. Trust in God. He is my rock and salvation. He will not leave me alone." Then he thought for awhile and whispered, "That the path will be a quick one." He pointed upward. I asked if he was referring to the path to heaven and he nodded. Then he whispered, "Just get me there." He lifted his hand, made a soft fist and punched the air. I asked if this meant he wanted a direct route to heaven and he nodded. He pointed his finger in a figurative circular route and smiled. We prayed for his intention. Michael was noticeably tired and his eyes closed.

My last visit with Michael was just after his doctor told him there was nothing more to be done for him except to keep him comfortable. He was crying and I wiped his tears. I said, "I'm sad, too. But I'm happy for you, too. You've definitely told Jesus just how you feel. I know He hears you." I prayed this powerful prayer:

> Jesus, I believe in You.
> Jesus, I love You.
> Jesus, I trust You.
> Jesus, I praise You.
> Jesus, I thank You.

I tearfully said good-bye to a tearful Michael.

The following morning, Michael died. Though I wasn't with him physically, I was with him in thought and spirit.

Michael taught me many lessons. He was a selfless man who never doubted his belief in God and that Jesus was his Savior. As I questioned my own capability of addressing his complex spiritual needs, I trusted that God put me with him because together we had something to offer each other, particularly being nourished by prayer. As I listened to what Michael was saying in his writing, art, music, and tears, I found a man with deep love for God and others. I acknowledged his sadness, his existential questions, his uncertainty, his need for others to visit him, and his extraordinary generosity of spirit and resources such as his life insurance policy. Michael delighted in small things like sitting in a chair instead of a bed. He never complained about his condition. We shared our emotions together whether we were laughing or crying. Curiosity and hopefulness were his constant companions.

A priest friend told me that theology is really about our own relationship with God. Thinking of that, I thought how well Michael understood theology! He trusted God, wrote about Him, wanted to talk to Him and about Him. He loved the olive wood cross, which he showed by often holding it.

After my visits with Michael, my heart will never be the same. It is full of love and thanks for his friendship and his influence in my life. I believe we can spiritually communicate with those who've died, and I talk to Michael from time to time. I ask him to show me the way with complex patients, that I can be the chaplain I'm meant to be with particular patients, just as I was with Michael. Though I receive no actual words from him, our connection is alive.

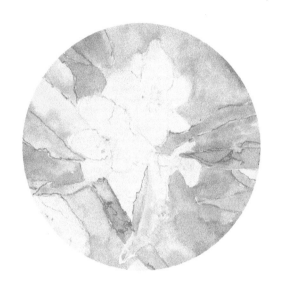

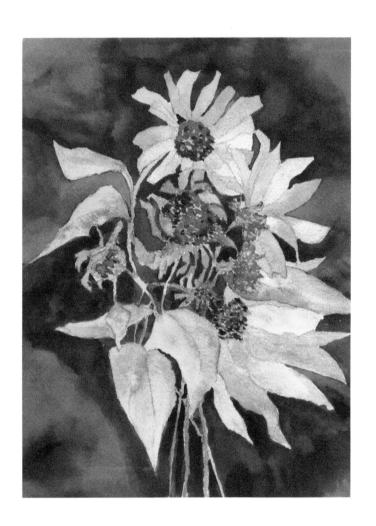

Brown-Eyed Susans

A dinner party bouquet
   two days before
   Brown Eyed Susans
   become a still life for my painter friend and me.

Once lifted heads of youth and grace
   bright
   vibrant
   shapely

Now nodded heads in reminiscence
   weathered
   twisted
   shriveled

"Like our lives," said my friend.
"Yes, our lives," I said,
"but still full of light within."

Ben
"I've gone from a pile of manure to a whole new world."

*B*en collapsed with heart failure. Since no comprehensive heart treatment was available in his state, he and his wife, Penny — for a heart patient must have a constant caregiver — made their home away from home for two years in our city, which hosts an internationally acclaimed heart center

Ben was imposing, handsome, dignified, vulnerable — and now, a heart failure patient. He described his transition from heart failure to a potential heart transplant like this: "I've gone from a pile of manure to a whole new world."

The day-to-day journey from the edge of death to a renewed healthy life is full of pitfalls and joys. Penny often communicated for Ben and for herself, and she recounted the monumental challenges she faced in her role: To be present each day in a foreign medical environment, digest information about unknown medical terms, witness the ups and downs of her husband enduring intensive procedures, and question what the final outcome would entail, I never saw her falter; she was with Ben every step of his journey.

Ben received a left-ventricular assist device, or LVAD — an elaborate, complicated electromechanical device designed to replace the function of his heart and serve as a bridge to his hoped-for transplant — which was implanted in his chest and connected to an external battery and monitor. He was hospitalized at first, then he and Penny moved into a temporary home in a nearby apartment. Eventually they received permission to return to their out-of-state home, where Ben would receive long-distance heart monitoring while they waited for a transplant, unsure of how long that would take. But severe complications necessitated an emergency flight transport back to the heart center, where Ben was placed on the top of the list for a transplant. Meanwhile, Penny, with the help of their children, moved into and furnished an apartment near the hospital that would serve as their long-term home.

Only days later the call came. A heart was immediately available. The cardiologist said, "You have five minutes to decide — do you want it, and are you ready?" Ben and Penny called their son-in-law doctor for advice, quickly prayed, then the phone rang again. "Yes or no?" asked the cardiologist. They drove to the hospital — which signaled a "Yes!" for a new heart.

In retrospect Ben recognizes he is still on the journey to wellness. "I'm not of out of the woods yet, but I feel blessed to have been given a second chance," he said. "The darkest time in the transplant process was when I was Life Flighted from Boise to Salt Lake due to complications with my LVAD. It was the fear of the unknown, of being backed into a corner. I had such feelings of despair about the seriousness of my condition; I wondered if it would compromise having a successful transplant. Leaving home and our family and friends again was difficult. It was a horrible time."

It's often said in the medical world that patients would never survive without a caregiver. Penny excelled in that role — 24/7 for two years. Ben said, "Her constant caring and undying love are the only reasons I'm on this earth."

After Ben's transplant and after he started his recovery, Penny openly talked of her feelings. "At first I was mad at Ben for not taking better care of himself and being in this position," she said. "I hated being away from home, especially living in temporary apartments. I missed our family and friends."

She continued, "One day I looked at him and thought, 'This poor man.' I had a change of heart — I was more understanding and patient and more focused on meeting the goals that would extend his life." She laughed but said it was so difficult to accept the challenges when she didn't know what a drive line was or how to give injections in Ben's stomach. She summed up her experience this way: "You find you do things you never thought you could do. You don't have a choice."

Support from family and friends helped to maintain Penny's spirit. Daily talks with their daughter, an email circle maintained by their friends, visits from out-of-town friends sharing dinners — each step supported Penny and ultimately Ben. One example: Ben, an alumnus of Gonzaga, planned to watch from his hospital room as the Zags played in the finals of a basketball tournament. His heart surgeon brought in Zag game gear including a foam mitt to wave. Lots of laughter and good will! The hospital heart support group — composed of heart patients and their caregivers — provided ongoing help and understanding, because as Penny says, "We're all in this together."

From a chaplain's view, Penny and Ben were easy to love. They were gracious and grateful to everyone. Ben's faith was evident. A life-long Catholic, he welcomed visits from me and others who provided spiritual care: Holy Communion, praying, listening. He welcomed prayer from the Carmelite sisters. He spoke of his mother in her 90s who called him 'Miracle Man' and prayed for him each day.

Penny's spiritual well-being centered on the practical: Whether Ben was walking or not walking, questioning if his medication cognitively impaired him, wondering how to cope with his discomfort in sleeping with this machine, his ability to swallow, speaking on his behalf to the medical team, arranging living quarters in a new city. Each of her actions demonstrated the spirit that was alive within her.

I asked Ben why he thought he was selected to receive a new heart. He said, "God only knows. Maybe he has a plan for me to do something else in life. I hope I recognize his plan and take advantage of this special gift of life. My relationship with God is different — stronger."

Since we were close in age, I wondered how I'd respond to an abrupt interruption in my life if my husband had been in Ben's situation and I'd have to care for him as Penny did for Ben. If that should ever happen to us, I have a script of love written by these two people. The love of Penny and Ben is based on complete trust, demonstrated by each of them fulfilling their separate roles. Ben's role was precisely following the instructions of his medical team. Penny's was to respond to Ben's every need—injections, monitoring, chauffeuring, listening, loving. Their love was strengthened in the face of seemingly impossible physical and emotional complications that swept them right to the edge of death. I was touched to see how their love included respect for each other and for every person who entered their realm.

The heart is a metaphor for life and love. The hearts of Penny and Ben brought new life to each of us. They brought life and love to their family, their friends, and to the larger community Ben served in elected office for many years.

As a chaplain, simply being present to witness this transformation of two people was the work of the spirit — not measurable, yet observable to those who journeyed with them. I became a different person by witnessing their transformation from broken to whole, from dispirited to spirited. I join with them in saying, "I am in awe."

—⁓——⁓——⁓——⁓—

The last time I saw Ben and Penny at the hospital was after their medical team had said it was safe to move from their Salt Lake apartment to their real home. Ben shuffled with his walker to their car, and Penny prepared to take the wheel. Nine months later, when I was in their city for the holidays, I asked if we could meet for coffee. I watched, awestruck, as driver Ben and passenger Penny emerged from their car and walked with great ease across the street. I was so caught up in my own surprise, I ran out of the door to greet them, hug them — so much had I missed them!

Ben talked freely of his meetings with Salt Lake doctors who visited their city for heart clinics. Such a bond had been formed. The long, tight hugs they shared with their doctors were normal to them — but looked at with surprise by local physicians. "When you have a life-and-death relationship with your doctor, of course you're going to hug!" said Ben with a laugh.

I was thrilled to hear about the new activities that filled their lives. An avid golfer, Ben has resumed playing, although he has "some work to do" to improve his game. The new governor of Idaho, a personal friend of theirs, asked Ben to be a member of his transition team and recommend people to fill posts in the governor's administration. Ben was also asked to emcee the governor's inaugural ball dinner.

Ben and Penny looked back at their medical journey, which he'd described as going "from a pile of manure to a whole new world." Penny beamed, "Now our story goes from hospital gown to tuxedo."

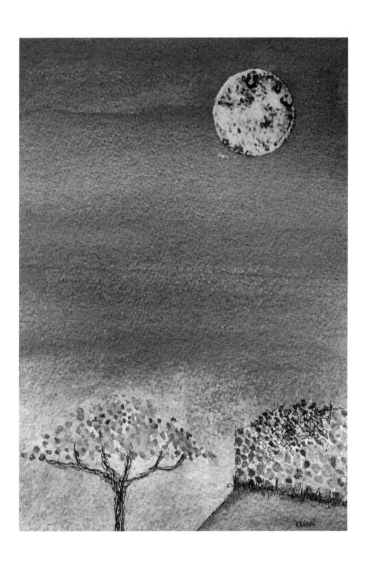

Spring Moon

New days sheltering in place—
solitude of someone else's making—
as hearts, bound and unbound,
attend to spring.

Tight purple plum buds
answer the sun's warm call
to live, expand, flower
explode in fushia and crimson

Lilacs billowing over our garden wall
beg a childhood memory
of my mother holding me tight
nuzzling our noses
in tiny star configurations
inhaling fragrant fullness.

In cold spring night
bulbous Flower Moon
majestically emerges over the mountaintop
to light pure darkness
connecting the universe
enveloping us in solidarity of beauty.

Linda
"I want to die. I miss my mom."

"*I* looked like a million bucks. Now I'm a crumpled mess." These were Linda's first words to me as I visited her in the rehab center of our hospital. Only 50 years old, she suffered a series of strokes that left her partially paralyzed on her right side and with a degree of brain impairment.

She said she had all the "right things" — a high-paying job at a big tech firm, a snazzy car, a beautiful condo, lots of friends, a loving family, and many good times. Now all of that was gone except for her loving sister, Terri, who took responsibility for Linda's care. Linda's hospital room looked as if an interior designer was at work. Family photos, hand-made quilts, a welcome wreath on the door, flower arrangements, bed linens — all contributed and arranged by Terri.

Among the family photos was one of their mother and her obituary framed with it.

"She died when I was here. I didn't even see her. Or go to her funeral. How do you think that makes me feel?" Linda asked.

"You must have felt alone," I said.

"More than that. I didn't even say good-bye. I still can't believe she is gone."

Linda's rehab progress was slow. Fitted with a leg brace, she could begin to take steps with a walker. Most of her time was spent in a wheelchair, which she could maneuver with one hand. Each time I visited Linda, I asked if I could pray with her, and she always said yes. I always asked what she wanted me to pray for and she almost always said, "Healing for me." Although she was Catholic, she didn't want to see a priest or even receive Holy Communion.

When Linda moved to a beautiful rehab center away from the hospital, I asked if I could visit her there. This was something I rarely did, but with permission from Linda and my supervisor, it seemed my visits may help her. In my first visit I said she must feel lucky to be in such a beautiful place.

"I don't feel lucky," she said. "I don't know what I'll do here. I'm living on borrowed time."

"What makes you say that?" I asked.

"Because I don't want to live."

Linda told me about her desire to be with her mother. We tearfully prayed, asking God to show

Linda the way. I asked if I could visit the next week and Linda said, "Of course."

The next week she began, "Everyone in this place wants to talk with me because I'm younger. Everybody else here is old. This isn't enough anymore."

"Where would you find something that is enough?"

"In heaven with my mother. I can't get there because my sister won't allow it. She said it's not my time to go. I have nothing to fall back on. No visitors. No one wants to see me because. . .I don't know why."

"Do you have some idea?" I asked.

"I think they think I'm on the last leg of my life. Or too embarrassed because they haven't come to see me."

"Did you think of calling them?"

"I don't really care if I see them or not."

"Would you call a friend in a similar situation?" I asked.

"Depends on how close I was to them. My best friend, Maria, left a few minutes ago. I can't take it anymore. I wish I could find a way around this. Not being able to get up to go to the bathroom. When I lost my right arm I thought I lost everything. I don't want to seem pretentious but I don't want to live this way. I want to go. I just don't care at all. Let me waste away. Give me some pills. I want to be remembered as a sweet girl who did lots of things for others."

The following Sunday Linda's blinds were open and she stared out the window from her bed. She accepted Holy Communion which I had brought her. Then she said, "I want to die. I miss my mom."

"Tell me what you loved about her." I said.

"She was sweet, Catholic, small, loved children."

"Do you talk to her?"

"I do but I don't get an answer. I'm not sure if she can hear me."

"Yes, she hears you," I said.

The next Sunday Linda immediately told me she'd made plans to end her life the following weekend. She said she thought she could trust me not to tell anyone. I told her I was obligated to tell her sister and the facilitator of the rehab center. She said I shouldn't be conflicted about supporting her plan. She wanted to be with her mother and this was the best way to do it. Simple as that. I asked if she'd like to see a priest and she said no. Nor would she receive Holy Communion. Then she asked me to bring her large doses of sleeping pills. I told her I couldn't be part of her plan. She said it wasn't necessary for me to visit her again.

I called her sister. Terri knew of Linda's request for pills and of her plan to end her life. She told me Linda was seeing a psychologist who was aware of her situation. She was also taking antidepressants. Terri asked me to visit again because she said Linda always talked positively about my visits.

The following week I dropped by near lunchtime. Linda was in the dining room slouching in her wheelchair at a table with an elderly woman. Linda looked at me. Listlessly she said, "Oh, hi."

"I'll help you in any way I can." I said.

"No, you won't. It's not necessary to visit again."

When she wouldn't engage with me, I turned and walked away feeling inadequate.

As I explained this visit to Terri, she said Linda was like this to everyone. She just wanted to be alone. I asked if I could write to her and Terri said that would be fine.

I wrote brief notes and enclosed prayers. Terri said Linda opened the first few notes but refused to open the others. Terri did open them and read them to her. She said Linda was indifferent.

Linda made a conscious choice not to eat and little by little she succeeded in dying.

Terri called me the morning after Linda died. I prayed for her eternal peace with God in the company of her mother. I attended the viewing for Linda, packed with extended family and friends. Many framed pictures of Linda in younger days were everywhere — and the way she'd described herself was accurate. She did look like a million bucks. Her body was in an elaborate rose-colored casket with pink flowers in hundreds of varied shades surrounding her. Linda's immediate family laid her to rest next to her mother the following day in a private graveside ceremony.

To be a chaplain is to be a companion in the journey of life. With Linda I felt my companionship was inadequate. The day she said it wasn't necessary for me to visit again, I wept from my sense of failure and for Linda, who was feeling so diminished. I had to trust and respect her for making the decisions she made about excluding people from her life including me. But that exclusion — the end of our companionship — was painful.

The soul and the body are one; they cannot operate independently. So why should I feel that the tugging at my stomach is also not a tugging at my soul? The density and heaviness of sorrow is a body-and-soul connection. Linda must have felt this tugging within herself, too.

When I think of Linda, I'm reminded of Rilke's lines:

We are only the rind and the leaf.
The great death that each of us carries
   inside us is the fruit.
Everything enfolds it.

Linda has shown me the fruit.

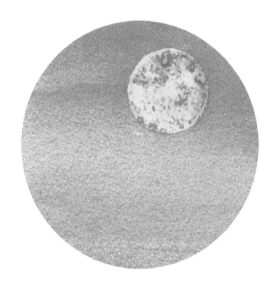

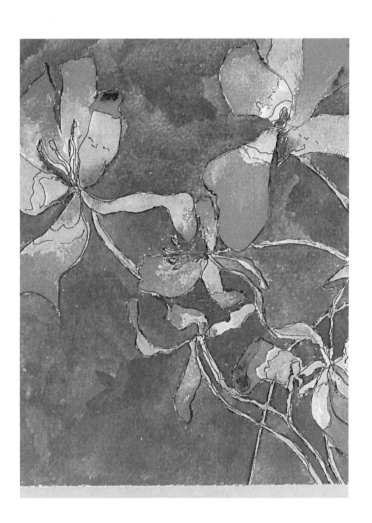

Tulips

Garden fresh
spring red tulips alive with rain drops—
a bouquet on our kitchen table.

Moment by moment, day by day,
nature works.

Six petals of each
        tightly enveloped
        suddenly burst
        change to orange and gold --
        refined cusps of brilliance
        to thin, twisted, hanging flower parts—

        life to death.

Bulbs,
secure and patient in the earth,
wait for the next life
of red spring tulips.

In the company of tulips,
are we
dying and being born?

John
"I believe in the promise of eternal life in the scripture. What if it's not true?"

"*I* always knew John would die but I could not admit it."

But when he did die, nothing prepared me for the sadness.

Nothing prepared me for the peace.

A text from our social worker as I arrived home from the hospital brought the news of John's death. Sitting at our kitchen table, hunched in grief, head in hands, I wept, sobbed, moaned, gasped. Then I stopped. I thanked God that John was at peace. This wasn't about me. It was about a man with the highest hopes of success in a complicated heart process. It was about a man who is loved by his beautiful and faithful wife and family. It was about a man with friends in our hospital's heart community who loved and supported him. In the end it was about a man with a depleted body that could no longer carry on. It was about a man who was at peace with saying goodbye to this world and embracing the next.

Fifteen months earlier, John was in the hospital at Christmas time. Connected to an IV pole and with many visible ports on his neck and arm, he was sitting in a chair near a large picture window that enveloped a view of the imposing snow-covered mountains with the morning sun streaming in. He was being kept alive on an LVAD, a surgically implanted device that kept his heart functioning while he waited for a transplant. He motioned me over to him.

Through his coughing, he said, "Better to be sitting in the sun coughing my guts out than sitting in bed." He paused. "I don't know what to do about my life." He paused, then continued. "I believe in the promise of eternal life in the scripture. But what if it's not true? I want to be here, to do so many things with my family. But you know, I'm not sure I will be here. Still, I've provided for Rita if something should happen to me."

He paused a long time. "But I'd rather be here doing things with her," he said with a laugh.

In a room full of Christmas decorations and messages of love from family and friends, John continued. "Have you met my family?"

"Yes, I've met Rita many times, your parents,

your in-laws. I saw your fishing friends and other heart patients with you."

"You understand. Am I wrong in wanting to stay? It's eleven months since my LVAD surgery. Then it was lung surgery, a serious infection, a leg injury, and now dialysis! Failing kidneys!" He threw up his hands. "My body just dives. I can't even pee the right amount."

The nurse came in with meds and applesauce for him to take with the meds. John put the spoon to his mouth. His hand was shaking. "See that? It shakes like that all the time. I can't even write a text."

He pointed to two books given him by the heart group. "They're supposed to be really good, but I can't read them. Focus. I can read for a second, but I can't understand what I read. I can't believe it. I was never like that. What should I do? My doctor says I can make it through this, but I don't see it happening. Where is God?"

I said I knew he always talked about his belief in God and the afterlife. It was only recently that he had questions. I suggested that he love the questions. To return to his original beliefs and talk to God about it. I asked if he'd like an example of what that talk might sound like. John nodded.

I said, "Dear God, right now I have a lot of questions about You and the afterlife. I thought

I knew what I believed but there are so many questions in my life, and now I'm unsure. Listen to me, please. Help me to know You are with me. Thank you, God."

John was silent, then said, "I know. I need to talk to God instead of questioning all the time."

The doctor and respiratory therapist came into John's room and I left.

Two days later John was sitting in a chair opposite his wife Rita, who was sitting on his bed. She patted the bed next to her for me to sit.

John said, "I'm so sad and depressed at the extent of this condition. I don't see the way that I'll improve enough for a transplant."

Rita added, "There are a lot of complications. I'm not dismissing the seriousness of his condition. I think we could use a prayer."

Together we held hands and leaned toward each other. I began, "Dear God, I lift John and Rita up to you and thank you for the gift they are to so many in our world. Bring your healing presence to John and Rita in mind, body, and spirit. Thank you for the medical staff who minister to John each day. Help them to bring their very best skills to him. Show John and Rita the way in this journey of life. Strengthen their faith in You, dear God, and the promise of eternal life you have made to those who believe in You. Dear God, we believe in You, trust in

You, praise You, love You, and thank You. Amen."

Rita held John's hand, turned to him, and said, "You need to do what's best for you. I will always love you. I'll miss you if you're not here. I want whatever will bring you peace."

John mournfully replied, "I know. But what if there's nothing more than a flower pot at the end?"

I encouraged, "John, remind yourself of the teachings you've learned all your life. Trust me. Do you think a loving and compassionate God is going to leave you with a simple flower pot?"

He laughed. "It does sound ridiculous."

"When you don't know what to say, just say, 'Jesus, I love You.' That will be all you need."

"I know. But will I remember?" asked John.

"Yes, I think you will." I said. "In case you forget, just say the name of Jesus."

John was in and out of the hospital during the next few months. For long stays in the hospital, Rita parked their RV in the hospital parking lot. One day when John was alone in his room, he told me, "Rita needs her space. You can't live with this stuff every minute."

Most times I visited with John, Rita was with him. I prayed with them. The existential question continued to concern John. With every assurance that God was with him, I prayed that his faith would become stronger.

Starting with my initial impressions of John, his wide welcoming smile, his bright gray engaging eyes, his easy manner and funny quips, I understood why he was loved by so many. He and Rita welcomed visitors even when John was sickest. They listened and commented positively to those who had successful LVADs and heart transplants, though it must have wounded them that John wouldn't walk that path. They continued to hope even in moments of despair.

Fifteen months after our Christmastime conversation, in the final days of John's life, he was sedated so his ventilator could provide the oxygen he needed. One morning Rita and I met with our palliative care doctor. Rita had many questions and the doctor responded with concrete answers. The conclusion was clear: Hope was running out. Rita said John was emphatic that he didn't want to be kept alive with artificial means. She said she needed to talk with her children. She asked me for a copy of the notes I was writing. She wanted to make sure she had the right information to share with the family.

"What are you thinking you'll say when you talk to them?" I asked.

"They'd appreciate my being clear," she said. "We've spent 20 years in and out of the hospital.

Often, we didn't tell them what was going on. John has had serious hospital stays in the past years but he bounced back."

"It would take very little to cause a complication or a setback in this situation," the doctor said. "Really, what the whole situation reflects is just how frail his body is. Influenza A is not a serious infection in and of itself, but it could have a serious impact on his body because he has little reserve."

"What can we do for you, Rita?" I asked.

"Just what you've done. Being kind and gentle as I've tried to accept this whole thing. Looking at death as inevitable," she said with tears in her eyes.

The doctor said, "Yes, this is what it means to have a terminal illness."

We prayed together and asked for guidance with the decisions of this day.

The following morning Rita and her daughter were at John's bedside. His face was covered with his ventilator mask, which was secured around his head and neck. He raised his arms in soft flailing and tried to move the mask. His nurse said there was an order to continue the sedation. Rita asked for a prayer for their family. Laying our hands on John, I asked for God to wrap this family in His love, for His merciful compassion in giving John rest and peace. When we finished, Rita said, "Yes, that is just what he needs — rest and peace. I love his soul."

Later that day John's stats continued to decline. Taking a message from his body, John resigned himself to death and a new life. Too frail to go home to die, John took his last breath with his family gathered at his bedside.

In reflecting on my two-year journey with John, I thank God for the sacred gift John gave to me and many others to witness his life. Even when he was declining, he welcomed us. That's just who he was. Some specific experiences with John will always remain with me. His hearty laugh when he told me he met Rita at a dance. He said he didn't like to dance but liked to pick up girls and he picked the best! I told him I remembered him with lighted candles and prayer at my church and he said, "Wow! I never had that happen before." And I said that we guard against having favorite patients but he certainly has risen to the top of the list for many of us. He said in wonderment, "You know how great that makes me feel?" His was the heart full of love, his being full of light.

At the end, medication clouded John's thinking; his conversations were fragmented and often jumped from one thought to another. His questions about God and the afterlife were vastly different than his original statement of belief in eternity. I tried to restate his learned beliefs while recognizing his changing outlook, caused by the effects of his meds and his clinical decline.

I learned it's necessary to unite myself to God before I visit patients. In that uniting I hope I can be present with every patient while listening and reflecting. Although our faiths were different, John and I united on basic beliefs in God, Jesus, the afterlife, and prayer as an extension of self to the spiritual world.

The poet Rumi writes:

> Be a lamp, a light, a lifeboat or a ladder.
>
> Help some's soul heal.
>
> Walk out of your house like a shepherd.

My hope is that John's soul healed. My soul is more alive because of him.

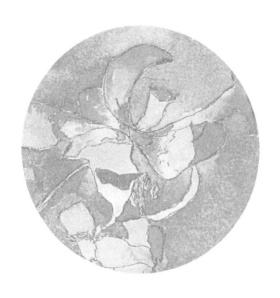

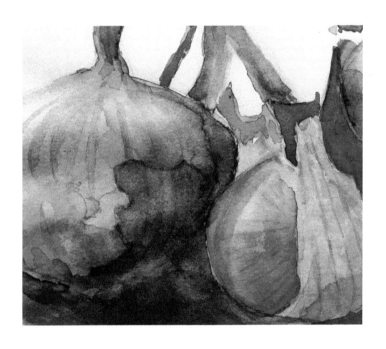

Layers

the doctor said
    we will withdraw life support
    the family would like you to pray with them

entering the room filled with quiet chatter
    two sisters approach me

please tell me about your sister I say

oh in the early days she
      laughed loved lived to the fullest
      then abuse abandonment alcoholism

generations gather quietly around the bed of Maria
    now comatose
    her face tattooed with three tears
    her knuckles with LOVE
    black roses on her arms
    a gold crucifix around her neck
    a spent depleted body

for what should we pray I ask
      peace
      that she knows we love her
      that her passage from this world is smooth
      that God welcomes her

    you may place your hands on Maria
    as we pray if you would like I say
    and gentle hands embrace her

I begin the prayer lifting Maria to God
      thanking Him for her presence in our lives

in this holy ritual of praying for the dying
      tears flow—
      tears of love, mourning, sadness
      of words unsaid, memories, peace --
      the layers of our deepest human expression

Jan
"Now my baby is dead."

My husband and I had just finished supper on a Friday evening when the phone rang. It was the hospital calling. A homeless woman had given birth to a stillborn baby, and she'd requested a chaplain visit. My husband asked if I wanted him to drive me to the hospital. He'd never done that before, and I accepted his offer.

The woman, Jan, was holding the baby in a crocheted blanket and cap in her small hospital room. I quietly introduced myself.

"Oh, take him," she yelled loudly and handed the baby to me.

"Sit here," she commanded as she slapped the bed near her. I sat and she lunged toward me, wrapped her arms around me and began to sob.

"He's dead. My baby is dead. I didn't even know I was pregnant. I'll name him after my father. My dad died. I think he's in heaven. Will my baby be, too?"

I assured her that her baby would be in heaven.

"Yes!" Sobbing, holding on to me, her head on my shoulder. "He has to be in heaven with my father. Oh, where are my children?"

"I had my first when I was 15. I think he's in Seattle." She continued to sob, blew her nose, and continued. "I had a baby last year. He's in custody. What's wrong with me? I was pregnant and didn't even know."

"Didn't know?" I asked.

"I thought I felt something move inside me but then it stopped. Then the pain. And now my baby is dead."

Jan's nurse came in and said the nurses who helped deliver the baby were here and would like to visit. We welcomed these beautiful young nurses, each one sitting at the foot of the bed. They quietly comforted Jan and answered her questions. The baby weighed just over four pounds and was about five months in development. Jan again said she didn't know she was pregnant. The nurses told her the baby would be cremated and shared the name of the mortuary that would have the cremains. They said the hands and feet of the baby would be imprinted in plaster of Paris and would be given to Jan.

Jan said she wanted to name the baby after her father.

As this happened, Jan's friend, Danny, was sitting in a chair close by in the confined room. He was reading his phone, then looked up and nodded to me. His gear, tents, backpacks, guitar, skateboard, and boots were stashed by the wall.

Jan asked me to pray with her. She said she was Catholic but she hadn't practiced for many years. She asked that I pray for her baby to be in heaven and to be at peace. I agreed to pray and invited Danny to join us at the bed. He came to the other side of the bed and bowed his head. The nurses placed their hands on Jan and on me during the prayer. I was still holding the baby. I prayed in the Catholic tradition, using familiar prayers, and both Jan and Danny joined in. I personalized the prayer with the baby's name and Jan's and Danny's names as we asked for God's protection of them. Then, in thanksgiving for the nurses, I prayed for them and their physical care and ministry to Jan.

When we finished praying, Danny returned to his chair. The nurses told Jan they'd take the baby when Jan was ready. She began to wail, saying she didn't know what to do. She said she had to see her baby again and I gently handed him to her. She took the cap off and opened the blanket; she cried more and kissed the baby's hands, feet, and face. She said nothing about the thin red scabs covering the protrusions on the baby's head, chest, arms, legs, and feet. Jan continued crying as she wrapped her baby and handed him to the nurse. The nurse placed him in a rolling wire basket, gently covered him with another blanket and quietly left the room.

Jan clung to me, continued to sob, and talked almost unintelligibly. I held her in my arms without doing or saying anything. In a few minutes she calmed down and lay back in bed. For the first time she was breathing more easily.

Caught up in the immediacy of my initial interaction with Jan, I'd had little time to observe. When I looked around, this is what I saw.

Jan was wearing a dirty and stained cami and hospital shorts. She was dirty — street dirty — with crusted dirt in her nails and knuckles. Her short, spiked, dirty hair was colored purple. Silver rings pierced her eyebrow and nose. Her face, stained from tears, was unwashed. She smelled, not only from being emotionally spent and delivering a baby, but from being unwashed and living on the street. Danny, too, was unwashed and dirty. His packs near the wall were worn and stained.

I told Jan and Danny I could stay as long as they'd like, but they seemed to prefer that I not linger. Danny said he was hungry and told Jan to call the cafeteria. She immediately picked up the phone and dictated exactly the food Danny said he wanted. When I told them I'd leave, Jan asked if I could come back the next morning. I agreed to see her then.

On the drive home, I told my husband as much as I could about the visit. I was tearful at the total sadness of the situation. This young street mother knew she wanted a connection to God for her baby, for herself. Yet she was oblivious to the fact that she was pregnant. Her smell became my smell because we had been so physically connected in hugging and crying. When we got home, I stripped off all my clothes in the laundry room, tossed them in the washer, and took a long shower. I cried through this shower — for Jan and her baby, for the homeless who line our streets and parks, for the unsolvable questions of What? How? Why? which I couldn't answer. I slept restlessly, paced during the night, and tried to make sense of what I'd experienced with this broken, sad young woman.

Saturday morning, I left home and told my husband that after I visited the hospital I would run a few errands. When I stepped off the hospital elevator onto the maternity floor, Danny was in a loud verbal altercation with two hospital security guards. His belongings were near him: backpacks, skateboard, and rolled tarps. He looked at me and said, "Hi, Rosemary." I told the guards I'd visited Danny and Jan the previous night. A third security guard approached us, and I told him who I was and my purpose for being here. He said he'd walk with me to Jan's room.

As we went down the hall, I could hear Jan screaming. The guard said the couple had a savage argument before I arrived; that was why they were escorting Danny out of the hospital. He said several people were trying to calm Jan.

As I stepped into the room, Jan screamed, "Rosemary! I want to die. The f---ing bastard is f---ing my best friend!" I stepped close to her bed and she reached out and held me tight around my waist, her head buried in my chest. I hugged her and said nothing.

"I want to die. But I love him. Tell him he can come back. F--- him."

"You want him back?

"They think I'm on drugs. I don't do meth and cocaine. I do smack and spice sometimes. Why did he do this with my best friend? F---ing my best friend. I want to die. I don't know what to do."

Jan began to calm down. I turned to see four others in the room with us: a doctor, a social worker, and two nurses. I also saw food all over the room, on the walls, floor and bed, the aftermath of an apparent food fight. The doctor quietly said they were transferring Jan to a clean room. I spoke with Jan and soothed her; she continued to hug me, cried softly and repeatedly said she just wanted to die. A wheelchair was brought and we took her to another room.

On the way, the nurse whispered to me asking if I could talk Jan into taking a shower. She hadn't showered since she checked into the hospital. When I suggested it, Jan agreed to shower and wanted razors, which she could not have. While in the hot shower for ten long minutes, she sang at the top of her lungs. It was a love song about always loving her man no matter what he did. Toward the end of the shower, she called to me and asked if I would wash her back. As she opened the shower door, I saw her back covered with open sores. I washed her back gently but thoroughly with a washcloth and soap. Jan dried and dressed in a clean hospital gown, pants, and socks. An aide put salve on the open sores.

When Jan was finishing dressing, her nurse told me Jan would be admitted to the psych unit because of her behavior and her stated desire to end her life. Her nurse asked for my help in talking with Jan about staying in the hospital.

Jan climbed into a clean bed, combed her hair and was calm. She asked for the wooden box that held the imprints of her baby's hands and feet. She calmly and gently held them and kissed them and put them back in the box. She began to talk about her life. She was 26, she said, and she'd done nothing with her life since her mother died some years ago. Living with Danny on the street was better than the shelter. They weren't married and couldn't sleep together in the shelter. Pitching a tent on the street was better for her. She knew she was bipolar but she refused to take medication that had once helped her. Illicit drugs were everywhere, she said.

I told Jan she'd remain with us in the hospital for a while. She continued to say she wanted Danny with her no matter what he'd done with her friend. I told her he wasn't able to return to the hospital at this time. She seemed resolved. Shortly, Security came with a wheelchair and Jan stepped quietly over and sat down. Covered with a warm blanket, the box of her baby's imprints on her lap, Security, her nurse, and I walked with her as she was wheeled to the psych unit. Jan didn't talk but reached for me as we entered the unit. I bent over and hugged her. She cried softly, thanked me, and turned away.

In the walk back to the maternity unit, the nurse told me the baby had been deceased for some days in utero. During that time period the baby had most likely been moving but with no nourishment.

That had caused the thin red scabs that covered his body. Eventually the natural response of Jan's body caused pain and led to the baby's eventual delivery. The nurse, young and kind, thanked me for my help with Jan.

From the hospital I went home, stripped all off my clothes and took another long, hot shower. I was totally sad for Jan, her struggles, her diagnosis, the conflicts in her life, her detachment from her previous children, her undetected pregnancy, and her delivery of her stillborn son.

During my visits with Jan, I thought I was being helpful, but I was tight and anxious. After the visits, when I breathed deeply, an overarching feeling of sadness encompassed me. It was such deep sadness that I cried after both visits and continued to cry for many days when I thought about Jan. I had never experienced any response like this in my life as a chaplain. It frightened me because it was so unlike me. This experience saddened me to the core.

The week after these visits, I arranged for a silent retreat at the Carmelite Convent. I wept in the silence of that first afternoon. I asked God to help me sort my feelings about my heartbreaking encounter with this lost, lonely, sad, disturbed girl. I reviewed my visits with her in my mind, wrote about them, prayed about them. I questioned myself about how I'd ministered to Jan. I wrote these words: held—hugged—kissed—cried—examined—loved questioned—lifted—exhaled—prayed—wept—sobbed

In this simple exercise of writing the action words of my encounters with Jan, I began to heal. I sketched a mother-child from a prayer book. I re-read Henri Nouwen's Wounded Healer about "binding my own wounds so I would be ready for the moment needed." Pope Francis says we must be so close to the sheep that we smell like them. I did smell like Jan, but I didn't linger in her smell — I'd changed and washed my clothes and showered. I wondered: Was that really being with the sheep as Pope Francis suggested?

I thought of the spiritual metaphors of this visit: prayer and the Spirit being with us, water as it cleansed Jan and changed her demeanor from harshness to softness, crying as we mourned the dead in our expressed sadness.

I thought of my own daughters and how observant they were of every aspect of pregnancy and how protective they were of the baby they carried. I wondered what it was that tipped Jan to her life. The death of her mother? Her unmedicated bipolar disorder? Her depression? Her loneliness? A combination of these? I thanked God for Jan and what I had learned from her. I prayed for her peace and reconciliation.

After three days of silence, I found renewal, cleanliness, a shift from sadness to reconciliation. The morning of the final day of the retreat I woke. The world seemed peaceful, still, and quiet. In the darkness of the night, eight inches of fluffy snow had fallen. The blanket of snow resembled the blanket we'd draped over Jan as she left the maternity unit. It was a sign of transition, of renewal, of my own renewed peace and quiet...and the blessing of being able to carry on.

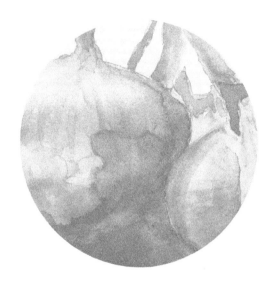

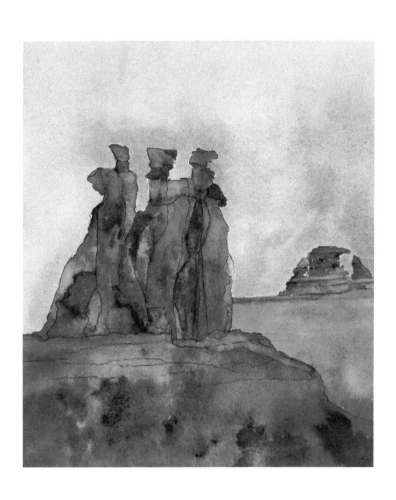

Utah Red Rock Formation

Some say the three gossips
I say we three sisters
   Barbara
   Mary Ellen
   Rosemary
towering
colorful
unified
withstanding storms
in solidarity
unforgettable
indestructible
steadfast
faithful
strong
   present in our world

JoAnn
"I feel very humbled...All I know is that I needed help and it came."

When I was on the hospital's neuro rehab floor visiting a patient, I stepped into the empty exercise room to make a phone call. Out of the corner of my eye I saw a patient with two physical therapists. Suddenly I realized the patient was a longtime colleague. She was struggling to walk in a straight path. She sat on the side of some exercise equipment. I neared the therapist and whispered that the patient was a friend. She said I could talk with her.

"JoAnn, it's Rosemary," I said. I felt the need to tell her because I remembered she'd been diagnosed with macular degeneration.

"I know who you are," she said.

"When you're finished here, may I visit you?"

"Yes. They'll tell you the time. I'm trying to get used to this schedule."

JoAnn. I thought about her. Our lives had some parallels. We were both retired educators who had embraced second careers. Hers was serving as mayor of a small city for 32 years, being reelected seven times. She was involved in numerous community affairs and specialized in conflict resolution. And as a pillar of the community, she served on many significant boards. We were both Catholic but attended different parishes. We collaboratively worked on a nationally acclaimed project — 3Rs: Rights, Responsibilities, Respect — which helped to address the multicultural issues and interpersonal relationships we faced in our own educational settings and in our ever-changing community.

Later that afternoon, I visited JoAnn. Three friends were with her and her room was full of bouquets of flowers. JoAnn was sitting in a chair. She said, "I had a stroke."

"A stroke?"

"Yes. I'd just finished my taxes when something went wrong. I knew it was serious. I went to find Daisy." Daisy lived in an adjoining apartment and was one of the three people now visiting. Daisy called 911, and within minutes, JoAnn was brought to the best stroke treatment hospital in the intermountain west. JoAnn was scanned, diagnosed, then assigned to rehab. Her neurological damage was treatable. She'd be in rehab for a few weeks.

We continued an easy conversation. I asked JoAnn if she would like me to pray with her and she agreed — and said I should pray not for herself but for all families. I invited her visitors to join us and we extended our hands in a circle as I prayed. I prayed as JoAnn requested but also included thanks for the friends who were with her, who continued to support her. I prayed for those who ministered to her in our hospital — every person because there was no unimportant job. And I thanked God for JoAnn and the gift she is to our world. By the end of the prayer, everyone was sniffling and the only man in the circle asked, "Am I the only one who needs a tissue?" We laughed.

"May I visit you again?" I asked.

"I hope you do," said JoAnn.

In rehab the daily schedule is noted on the board in each patient's room. There's always a full schedule and little time for lunch and rest. Therapy in its different forms — physical, occupational, and speech — is the reason patients are in the unit. In visiting JoAnn, I always asked if she was too tired from her therapy. "You are my therapy," she said. I never stayed long but always prayed with her. And always, when I asked what her intention for our prayer should be, she never mentioned herself, but always wanted to pray for others.

I once asked her if she'd like to see a mutual friend. She did and I invited Martha, also an educator who was connected with our work in the 3Rs. We arranged a time before JoAnn's lunch.

"Oh, hello, darling!"

"It's been too long," said Martha.

Both were crying and both hugged for a long time.

"Well, this is a different way of getting attention," said Martha jokingly.

"Well, I got my taxes done. Then I realized something was wrong."

"How did you know what to do?"

"I can't believe my mind could pull it together — all the things that were happening — to say, 'stroke,'" JoAnn said, massaging her head. "I live in a two-story old house. And Daisy lives downstairs. She did it. Here, I have whatever I need."

"What helped you the most?" Martha asked.

"God has been with me. I can't tell time. I don't know east from west. I'm not able to read. I try to follow the news on TV. And they tell me I can recover."

How are you feeling about all of this?"

"I feel very humbled. It could have been so much worse. All I know is that I needed help and it came. My nephew is an attorney and got all the wheels turning. It just works its way like a great yeast."

Martha asked about JoAnn's family and JoAnn began to talk of them but became confused with the layers of family and their respective places. "I guess I'm having trouble with this — thinking and trying to remember," JoAnn said. "The night this happened, those from the hospital board who served with me were right here beside me." She named prominent people. "All I can say is 'Thank you and I'll work hard to get better.'"

There was a pause, then JoAnn said, "Can't tell time? Damn. That's going to be hard. And I'm going blind. But I can hear music, thank goodness. Can't follow books on tape. Other things will come, thank God." She talked about going to the Senior Center and she's grateful for the "chefy things" prepared for her and for the support of her friends.

Lunch arrived which was our cue to end our visit. The usual hugs and love were extended, and Joann said good-bye to both of us.

A few days later JoAnn was going home. I asked if I could visit her before she left and she said yes.

"What is most important to you now?" I asked.

"Being open to all that is and can be, the beauty that is all around me, the peace that is possible, and the commitment we have to each other. And there is the love I have of the Trinity... different depths.

Superficiality has no place. The love of God is above everything."

"Even after your stroke this is the most important?" I asked again.

"Yes. The cry is louder. I want to listen. It's never a little. I have to figure how it can be used in God's way. We must love more and more especially those who've been damaged. I grew into being bigger than I am."

"How does prayer work for you?" I asked.

"Private conversations with God. Finding ways of finding 'What is.' And to cleanse myself. With this stroke I lost my capacity to speak the same way but it's returned in some ways. It's deeply rooted in who I am. It just is. Maybe God blessed me and said, 'Keep up the good work, honey!'" And she laughed.

"What do you most want to have happen now?"

"I want to take time to breathe, ingest beauty, have time for a little child," she thoughtfully said.

We said goodbye with the promise of another visit soon.

JoAnn was open, willing to share her vulnerabilities. I felt in awe of her, proud of her as a friend, and nourished by her unflinching belief and trust in God. After each visit I was lifted in spirit. My usual response when I visit a stroke patient is sorrow for their condition and feeling secretly thankful I wasn't the one who suffered the stroke. With JoAnn it was as if she was giving a gift in her condition, a gift of faith, a gift of love, a gift of looking at things differently and more positively.

I asked myself: Why was it JoAnn and not me? We're close in age. Will this happen to me? Would I respond in the philosophical and theological ways JoAnn did? Or would I whine about my condition? Would I think God didn't love me or would I think God loved me even more, like JoAnn thought? JoAnn didn't once falter in her belief and trust in God, but instead took strength from her medical challenges.

JoAnn struggled with cognitive functioning but was aware of her shortcomings. She realized that words didn't come easily to her. She knew she wasn't coherent in thought. But she didn't lament those losses. She didn't wish it wasn't so. Even before her stroke she knew of her macular degeneration. She accepted her diagnosis and willingly participated in therapy. She was successful enough to be discharged home.

In a few months Martha and I visited JoAnn in her home. Fresh from the beauty shop she looked very together even though connected to oxygen. She welcomed us and said she really needed this visit. She has had four or five strokes since the first. I asked her how she knew. "Something just doesn't connect like it used to," she said pointing to her forehead plus her continued inability to find words she said as she waved her hands. Increased macular degeneration precluded reading and watching TV. She tries to listen to the radio news but becomes distracted. Music is her solace.

Daisy lives with JoAnn. "Without Daisy I'd be dead," JoAnn quipped. Martha asked how we could help her. Without hesitation, "Get together every so often, listen to me, plan something that doesn't require much on my part but allows me to be part."

"Would you like to pray before we leave?" Pulling her chair close to us, she extended her hands to ours. We formed a close circle, heads bowed. JoAnn prayed, "That everyday we find the one person who needs us and communicate that that person is loved. Don't give up but give in with your heart." We all emerged teary but renewed.

I told JoAnn that I was writing the story of some of my patients including our meeting at the hospital. The identity of most patients was masked. Would she also like me to mask her or tell her story with her name and real conditions? In her no-nonsense way she said, "Tell it like it is. If I can help someone, then good."

Not one time in our visit did JoAnn bemoan her condition. It was never about her but about how grateful she was, praising those who help her and thanking God for the blessings of each day. I asked God to help me be more like JoAnn.

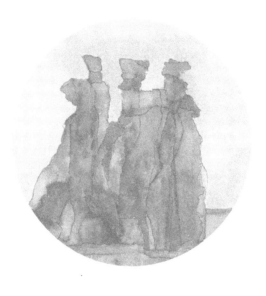

Afterword

When I was compiling the final edits to this book, God had one more lesson to teach me.

My brother-in-law, Dan, died in Virginia and as the eldest in the family who would attend his funeral, I was invited to give the eulogy. I was honored to be invited.

My sister, when she found out about Dan's death, said, "I feel like there is a hole in my heart." When I asked her what she meant she replied, "It makes me realize our own mortality. Our generation is dying." She, living in a very distant state, wasn't able to attend the funeral because of her own health issues.

My husband and I traveled to Virginia without problems. The day of the funeral, our family greeted friends and colleagues of my brother-in-law at the church where he and my deceased sister had been long-time parishioners. During the Mass, however, I became aware of an increased heaviness in my left side, as if I had ten pounds inside my chest. I straightened up, breathed deeply, and whispered to my husband that I felt faint. He gave me water to sip, which helped a little, but the pain didn't go away. When it came time for the eulogy, I felt quite ill, prayed I'd be able to deliver it just as I'd planned and practiced. I wanted to honor Dan and all of our family. I quietly walked to the place in the sanctuary and delivered the eulogy just as I'd hoped. Given the still heavy weight in my chest, I knew a divine presence supported me. After the funeral, the process of farewell to Dan was completed with a reception and then burial with military honors. At the end, I was exhausted.

When my husband and I returned to our hotel, I decided I had to rest, but as the intensity of the chest weight increased, I knew I needed to get to the hospital. My husband and son rushed me to the nearest place. Emergency department personnel responded quickly and expertly and within in an hour I was admitted to the hospital. Blood analysis showed abnormalities relating to my heart. Since I'd been healthy all my life, I was shocked. I told the doctor we had a family gathering that evening I needed to attend. Too, we had plane reservations the following day. Our intermountain city where the nationally recognized heart trauma center was located could help me. The ED doctor said, "I'm aware of your heart center. But you're not being discharged from this hospital until we determine what's happening with your heart and treat those symptoms!" For one who's used to making my own decisions, I was taken aback at the doctor's frankness and directness. I knew this was serious!

For four days I experienced life as a patient and received the most excellent care. The best news was that medication immediately relieved my pain and a series of heart tests and procedures indicated I'd had a mild heart attack. Doctor conversations and pharmacy directions provided the necessary focus.

Patient life is a busy life, just as it should be when medical attention is needed. But I had quiet times to reflect and think about why I was here. Not ever a TV watcher, the quiet was welcome particularly in the wee hours of the night. I found myself asking the same questions I ask my patients: What is most important to you? What do you need to take care of? What are you and God talking about? What needs to be included in your life that's not included now? What in your life can you now say "No!" to so you're opened to some other new opportunity?

I thought of the *Prayer for Healing*, developed by the Renew program, which has been a mainstay in my life for over 20 years.

Lord God, make me an instrument of your healing;
when I am weak and in pain, help me to rest;
when I am anxious, help me wait;
when I am lonely, help me to love;

when I place you apart from me, help me to
know that you are near.

Healing God, grant me not to demand
everything from myself,
as to let others help me;
nor to expect others to cure me,
as to do my own part toward getting better.
Grant me not so much to seek escape,
as to face myself and learn from the depths
of your love.

For it is in being uncertain and not in control
that we find true faith,
in knowing the limits of our mind and body
that we find wholeness of spirit,
and in passing through death that we find life
that lasts forever.

I have said this prayer hundreds of times, given
copies to friends, relatives and patients, and discussed its meaning in groups. I love this prayer. For
one who's always in charge and in control, the line
"For it is in being uncertain and not in control that
we find true faith, in knowing the limits of our mind
and body that we find wholeness of spirit" brought
me up short. Yes, this line was speaking directly to

me. Faith is that belief and affirmation in something far greater than I. It is Christ who is the universal presence, in tune with me and every other creature. It is my vulnerability that prompted a new insight, a new way of thinking. *The Gift Within*, I thought, was a perfect title for this book and message for me in my own journey of illness and recovery. I found a faith I hadn't recognized before. I talked with God in a way I hadn't done before. A mild heart attack brought me low and I thought of my life, my heart, in a different way.

This time provided some clarity and opportunity to formulate what is most important to me: continued spiritual development with focus on contemplation, enough time to ensure that I'm well and capable of participating in family activities, writing and studying with teachers who can lead me in the spiritual life, and, of course, meaningful chaplaincy service.

Sitting at my kitchen table a few weeks later, I told a friend what had happened to me at the funeral in Virginia. My friend commented on the significance of this event at this time in my life. "You did not have a perforated bowel. You had a heart attack." He said it wasn't coincidental that I was in the hospital receiving care for my heart at the very time I was writing a book about when I provided care for patients with heart-related issues, whether they were literal or spiritual. Could it be that my heart had been under attack by the pain and sorrow I've experienced in other people's lives and that only by the grace of God has my heart been watched over and tended, not broken, but reshaped for His purpose?

The heart! The very center of our being. When the heart begins beating, life begins. When a heart stops beating, life stops. When a heart is overwhelmed, it needs help. That is exactly what happened to me. I needed heart help and I received it with expertise and care. This experience made me stop, reflect, listen, pray, change. Yes, God is working in my life.

I've asked in conversations with my very ill patients, "Why?" Now it's my turn! I know how it feels to be vulnerable, to look within, to find something bigger than myself. I know what it means to talk to Christ and ask Him to show me the way for my life. I know more fully what my patients have been experiencing. I'm a better chaplain for that — for discovering the Gift Within.

Acknowledgments

To our patients, families and staff who shared their lives so generously with me, thank you.

To Reverend Lourduraj Gally Gregory for inviting me to his graduation from Clinical Pastoral Education and planting the seed to become a chaplain.

To Phil Cousineau, who asked, "Are you a writer?" With that question, he planted the seed that nurtured my "yes" to participate in Writer's Retreat in Connemara, Ireland. Once engaged in the writing process he stoked the fires of creativity with careful guidance and movement and helped me to find the gift within. Thank you.

To Rich Nash, editor, writer, mentor, encourager and friend. Thanks for saying that you were with me through the completion of this project, for helping me to think more like a writer and for suggestions for change when needed, and for your positive outlook — always!

To my fellow chaplain and friend, David Pascoe, sincere thanks for the conversations, clarifications, reflections and humor as we walk this journey as chaplains. The road is smooth with such a friend as you.

To my talented and wise art teacher, Marian Dunn, for your generous teaching and encouragement; to Patti Owen, the middle school art teacher who opened the door to art and friendship. Thank you.

To Peggi Blackman, Spiritual Care Volunteer Coordinator, supporter of spiritual services and a dear friend, thank you for your vision, support and friendship.

To Steve Sheffield for your original art on this book cover, thank you, for your inspiration and intuitive spirit.

To our children, Kathryn, Mary and Peter, with heartfelt thanks and love for your respect and honor of my work.

To my husband, Bruce, the sounding board, who has listened to hundreds of stories over dinner at our kitchen table and on long walks together, gratitude and love always.